Mindful Holistic Cleansing

Natural Remedies and pH Balance For Optimal Health

By Aidan Curtis

Are you looking to improve your overall health and well-being? Look no further! This book delves into the important topics of pH balance, the benefits of herbs and which herbs are best for the body, increasing energy, the power of fruit, parasites and detox cleansing, fasting, and meditation. Discover the impact that pH levels have on your body and how to maintain a healthy balance through the foods you eat. Learn about the various benefits of incorporating herbs into your diet, including improved digestion and immune system support. Increase your energy levels naturally with tips and techniques that will leave you feeling revitalized. Explore the power of fruit as a source of essential nutrients and antioxidants. Gain insight on the importance of parasite and detox cleansing for a healthier gut and overall well-being. Discover the benefits of fasting and how it can aid in weight loss and detoxification. And finally, learn the art of meditation and its ability to reduce stress, improve focus, and enhance overall mental and emotional health. With diverse viewpoints and practical advice, this book is a must have for anyone striving for a healthier and more balanced lifestyle.

CONTENTS

ALKALINE FOODS

The path to wellness and vitality lies in understanding the delicate balance of our body's natural pH levels. Alkaline foods are an essential cornerstone of this journey, offering a plethora of benefits that promote optimal health. By embracing a diet rich in alkaline forming foods, one can harness the power of nature's pharmacy and unlock a treasure trove of nutrients, minerals, and antioxidants. Alkaline foods are nature's gift to our health, offering a bounty of benefits that support our body's natural balance. These foods are rich in minerals, including calcium, magnesium, and potassium, which are essential for maintaining healthy pH levels in the body. By consuming a variety of alkaline forming foods, such as leafy greens, root vegetables, and certain fruits, we can help our bodies maintain a slightly alkaline state, which is optimal for overall health and well-being. The magic of alkaline foods lies not only in their nutrient density but also in their ability to support the body's natural detoxification processes. Our modern world is filled with environmental toxins and stressors that can disrupt our body's delicate balance. Alkaline foods act as gentle cleansers, helping to flush out these toxins and support the liver and kidneys in their vital roles. By incorporating alkaline-rich choices into our diet, we can enhance our body's natural ability to detoxify, leading to improved energy levels, clearer skin, and a stronger, more resilient body.

The road to good health is an enlightening journey, and having a grasp on the body's pH levels can be a powerful tool. Embracing a diet abundant in alkaline forming foods is a natural way to unlock a treasure trove of health benefits. These nature made medicines are rich in essential minerals such as calcium, magnesium, and potassium. The key players in this story are leafy greens, known for their vibrant hues and nutrient dense makeup. Think of kale, spinach, and Swiss chard, with their curly leaves and earthy flavors, ready to be transformed into delicious and nutritious meals. Root vegetables also have a leading role, with beets, carrots, and sweet potatoes adding a touch of sweetness and a plethora of benefits. Some fruits, like crisp apples and juicy lemons, are also part of the alkaline team, bringing a burst of flavor and a range of vitamins. By incorporating these natural, alkaline rich foods into daily meals, one embarks on a journey towards detoxification and vitality.

These foods support and enhance the body's natural processes, flushing out toxins that invade our modern world. It is a gentle yet potent path to wellness, resulting in increased energy levels and a strengthened, clearer body and mind. The journey towards wellness is an enlightening path, and understanding the body's pH levels is a powerful tool. Embracing a diet rich in alkaline-forming foods is a natural key to unlocking a treasure chest of health benefits. These foods, nature's true pharmacy, offer a bounty of minerals, with calcium, magnesium, and potassium in abundance. Leafy greens are the heroes of this story, with their vibrant colors and nutrient dense composition. Think of kale, spinach, and Swiss chard, with their ruffled leaves and earthy flavors, ready to be transformed into delicious, healthy meals. Root vegetables, too, play a starring role, with beets, carrots, and sweet potatoes adding a touch of sweetness and a wealth of benefits. Certain fruits, like crisp apples and juicy lemons, also join the alkaline team, bringing with them a burst of flavor and a host of vitamins. By incorporating these natural, alkaline rich foods into daily meals, one embarks on a journey of detoxification and vitality. The body's natural processes are supported and enhanced, flushing out the toxins that invade our modern world.

It is a gentle yet powerful path to wellness, with increased energy levels and a stronger, clearer body and mind.

Indulge in the mouth-watering taste and rejuvenating properties of alkaline foods. These powerful additions to our daily meals not only tantalize your taste buds but also ignite a symphony of sensations in our bodies. With each bite, we embark on a journey of detoxification and revitalization, as the flavors dance across our tongues and the nutrients nourish our cells. But the benefits of these foods go beyond just their delicious taste and nourishment. They also play a vital role in restoring our body's natural pH balance, creating a healthy internal environment. In a world filled with acidic foods that can lead to inflammation and other health issues, alkaline foods are a refreshing and vital counterbalance. And as we savor each delicious bite, we are not only pleasing our palate but also taking care of our body from the inside out. But the power of alkaline foods goes beyond just their physical benefits. They have a character-rich voice that speaks to our soul, evoking strong emotions and igniting a sense of overall well-being and vitality. These gentle yet potent foods support and enhance our body's natural processes, flushing out the toxins that threaten our modern world. And in return, we are rewarded with increased energy levels, a stronger, clearer body and mind, and a renewed sense of vitality.

So why settle for a bland and acidic diet when you can indulge in the flavorful and nourishing world of alkaline foods? Let their multiple senses and complex characters captivate you, and join us on a journey to ultimate wellness. With each bite, you are not just nourishing your body, but also satisfying your soul.

Incorporating alkaline foods into our daily meals is a wise choice for promoting overall wellness. Not only do these nutrient -rich foods add a burst of flavor, but they also play a crucial role in detoxifying and rejuvenating the body. By making these foods a regular part of our diet, we embark on a journey towards a stronger and clearer body and mind. These gentle yet potent foods support and enhance the natural processes in our body, aiding in flushing out the toxins that are prevalent in our modern world. The benefits of alkaline foods extend far beyond their delicious taste and nourishment. They also help to rebalance the body's pH levels, which are essential for maintaining good health. In today's society, our diet is often filled with highly acidic foods, which can lead to inflammation and various health issues. However, incorporating alkaline foods into our meals can have an alkalizing effect, neutralizing the acidity and promoting a healthier internal environment. By making these foods a regular part of our diet, we not only satisfy our taste buds, but also take care of our body from the inside out. This makes alkaline foods a valuable addition to any diet, promoting overall well-being and vitality.

Alkaline foods are renowned for their distinct and invigorating taste. They are a treat for the senses and can instantly enhance any meal. However, their appeal goes beyond just their flavor. These foods are also abundant in nutrients and offer a plethora of health benefits. From leafy greens to tangy fruits, alkaline foods not only tantalize the taste buds but also play a vital role in maintaining a healthy body. They are a perfect combination of deliciousness and nourishment, making them an excellent addition to any diet. Moreover, alkaline foods do more than just satisfy our palate and provide essential nutrients. In today's world, we are constantly exposed to harmful toxins from our surroundings, food, and even daily products. These toxins can accumulate in our bodies and lead to various health problems. However, by incorporating alkaline foods into our regular meals, we can support and boost our body's natural detoxification processes. This helps to eliminate toxins and leaves us feeling rejuvenated and refreshed. Alkaline foods offer a gentle yet effective way to detoxify and promote overall vitality. With increased energy levels and a stronger, clearer body and mind, they truly are a powerful path to wellness. So why not embark on a journey towards better health and add some alkaline foods to your daily meals? Your body will thank you for it

The effects of alkaline foods extend far beyond mere nourishment and flavor. These foods possess a gentle yet potent nature that can be felt through an increase in energy levels and a revitalized body and mind. Along with their delicious taste, they also aid in restoring the body's pH balance, a crucial aspect of overall health. In contrast to the modern diet, full of acidic foods that can cause inflammation and health issues, alkaline foods have an alkalizing effect that neutralizes acidity and promotes a healthier internal environment. By incorporating these foods into our daily meals, we not only delight our taste buds but also prioritize our internal well-being. They are a valuable addition to any diet, promoting overall vitality and wellness. In addition to their unique and refreshing taste, alkaline foods are renowned for their vibrant and tangy flavors. They provide a burst of sweetness and zest that tantalize the senses and leave a pleasant aftertaste. These foods are not just a treat for the taste buds, but also a source of essential nutrients and numerous health benefits. From leafy greens to citrus fruits, they are a vital component of maintaining a healthy body. Their flavorful nature is an added bonus that makes them an excellent choice for any diet. In summary, alkaline foods offer a perfect balance of taste and nourishment, making them an essential element in our daily meals. Their gentle yet powerful effects can be felt through increased energy levels and a stronger, clearer body and mind. Furthermore, their ability to restore the body's pH balance plays a significant role in maintaining overall health. Unlike the modern diet, which is high in acidic foods, alkaline foods have an alkalizing effect that counteracts acidity and creates a healthier internal environment. By incorporating these foods into our daily meals, we not only satisfy our taste buds but also prioritize our internal well-being.

This makes alkaline foods a valuable addition to any diet, promoting overall vitality and wellness. Known for their invigorating and refreshing taste, alkaline foods have a unique ability to tantalize your taste buds and leave a pleasant aftertaste. Their flavors are often described as vibrant and zesty, with a perfect balance of sweetness and tanginess. These foods are a delight to the senses and can instantly elevate any meal. However, their taste is not the only thing that sets them apart. They are also packed with essential nutrients and offer numerous health benefits. From leafy greens to citrus fruits, these foods are not only delicious but also crucial for maintaining a healthy body. The burst of flavor they provide is an added bonus, making them an excellent choice for any diet. Overall, alkaline foods are a perfect combination of taste and nourishment, making them an essential element in our daily meals. It's important to try to get fruit with seeds as much as possible the benefits of these fruits have an amazing impact on the bodies pH balance.

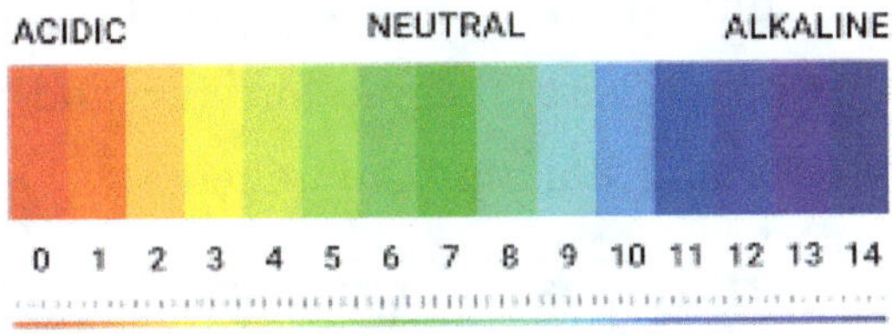

Examples of alkaline foods?

1. Leafy greens: These include spinach, kale, collard greens, and other dark, leafy vegetables.

2. Citrus fruits: Lemons, limes, grapefruits, and oranges are all high in alkaline-forming minerals.

3. Cruciferous vegetables: These include broccoli, cauliflower, and Brussels sprouts.

4. Root vegetables: Sweet potatoes, beets, carrots, and radishes are all alkaline foods.

5. Avocados: This versatile fruit is not only high in healthy fats, but it is also alkaline-forming.

6. Nuts and seeds: Almonds, cashews, chia seeds, and flaxseeds are all alkaline foods.

7. Garlic and onions: These flavorful ingredients are also alkaline-forming and offer various health benefits.

8. Fruits: Many fruits, such as apples, pears, and bananas, are alkaline-forming and provide essential vitamins and minerals.

9. Herbal teas: Certain herbal teas, like chamomile and ginger, are alkaline and can help balance the body's pH levels.

10. Plant-based proteins: Foods like tofu, tempeh, and legumes are all alkaline and make great alternatives to animal based proteins.

11. Coconut water: This trendy beverage is not only hydrating but also alkaline-forming.

12. Alkaline water: While it may be controversial, some believe that drinking alkaline water can help balance the body's pH levels.

13. Olive oil: This healthy oil is considered alkaline forming and can be used in cooking or as a salad dressing.

14. Spices and herbs: Many herbs and spices, such as turmeric, basil, and oregano, are alkaline and add flavor to dishes.

15. Seaweed: This nutrient dense food is also alkaline forming and can be incorporated into soups, salads, and sushi.

16. Moringa

17. Sea moss

18. Shilajit

19. Ginger

20. Coconut oil

Chapter Two

ACIDIC FOODS

While alkaline foods bring a plethora of benefits, their acidic counterparts can present challenges. Acidic foods, when consumed in excess, can disrupt the body's delicate pH balance, leading to a state of acidity within the body. This imbalance can trigger a cascade of unwanted effects, including inflammation and a range of health issues. From joint pain and digestive problems to weakened immunity and even contribute to the development of chronic diseases. The modern diet, with its abundance of processed foods, sugary treats, and carbonated drinks, tends to favor acidity. Foods like red meat, dairy products, and grains can be highly acidic, and when they dominate our plates, they tip the body's pH levels toward the acidic end of the spectrum. This acidic environment can become a breeding ground for unwanted bacteria and pathogens, causing further disruption to our health.

It is important to note that not all acidic foods are detrimental. Some, like lemons and oranges, are alkaline forming once consumed and offer a range of vitamins and minerals. However, the overconsumption of highly acidic foods can outweigh these benefits. The key to wellness lies in finding harmony between these two extremes. By reducing the intake of highly acidic foods and embracing the abundance of alkaline choices, one can strive for the optimal pH balance that the body craves. This balance is a delicate dance, and each meal presents an opportunity to tip the scales toward vitality and wellness. Thus with every bite a chance to write a new chapter toward a healthier future

Acid forming foods are those that, when metabolized by our bodies, leave an acidic residue. This can lead to a mucus forming and acidic environment in our bodies, which can have negative effects on our health. Meat, dairy, and processed sugar are all examples of acid forming foods.

Meat, especially red meat, is high in protein and fat, which when broken down during digestion, leave behind acidic by products. This can contribute to a buildup of acid in the body, which can lead to inflammation and other health issues. Additionally, the way meat is often produced, such as through factory farming and the use of antibiotics and hormones, can also have negative impacts on our health.

Dairy products, such as milk, cheese, and yogurt, also contain high levels of protein and fat. These can also leave behind acidic residues in the body. In addition, dairy products are often pasteurized, which can destroy beneficial bacteria and enzymes, making them more difficult to digest. This can further contribute to an acidic environment in the body.

Processed sugar, found in many packaged and processed foods, is another major contributor to acidity in the body. This is because refined sugar is quickly broken down and absorbed, leaving behind acidic byproducts. Consuming large amounts of processed sugar can lead to a range of health issues, including weight gain, inflammation, and an increased risk of chronic diseases.

While some foods are naturally acidic, our bodies have mechanisms in place to balance out and neutralize their effects. However, consistently consuming a diet high in acid forming foods, such as meat, dairy, and processed sugar, can overwhelm our body's ability to maintain a healthy pH balance.

There are, however, diverse viewpoints on the impact of acid forming foods on our health. Some argue that our bodies are naturally designed to handle acidic foods, and that the real issue is consuming too many processed and unhealthy foods in general. Others believe that it is not the specific foods themselves, but rather the overall balance of our diet, that is most important for maintaining a healthy pH balance.

In conclusion, while acid forming foods like meat, dairy, and processed sugar can have negative effects on our health, it is important to consider the bigger picture of overall dietary patterns and balance. Incorporating a variety of whole, plant based foods and limiting highly processed and unhealthy foods can help maintain a healthy pH balance and promote overall well being.

Examples of acidic forming foods:

1. 1.Sour cream

2. 2.White bread

3. Alcohol

4. 4.Coffee

5. Soda and other carbonated drinks

6. 6.Processed meats (sausages, deli meats)

7. Dairy products (milk, cheese)

8. Artificial sweeteners

9. Fried foods

10. 10.Refined grains (white rice, white pasta)

11. 11.Red meat (beef, pork, lamb)

12. Artificial preservatives and additives

13. High-fat foods (butter, margarine)

14. Chocolate.

Chapter Three

HERBS FOR HEALTH

Herbs have been used for centuries to promote health and well-being. These natural plants offer a variety of benefits for the body, both physically and mentally. From boosting the immune system to improving digestion, herbs have a lot to offer when it comes to overall health.

One of the main benefits of using herbs is their ability to support the immune system. Many herbs contain powerful antioxidants and anti-inflammatory compounds that can help prevent illness and fight off infections. For example, echinacea is known for its ability to strengthen the immune system and reduce the severity of cold and flu symptoms. Other herbs like ginger, turmeric, and garlic also have immune-boosting properties that can help keep the body healthy and strong.

In addition to supporting the immune system, herbs also have a positive impact on digestion. Many herbs have been traditionally used to aid digestion and improve gut health. For example, peppermint is known for its ability to soothe digestive issues such as bloating, gas, and nausea. Fennel and ginger are also commonly used to promote digestion and relieve stomach discomfort. By incorporating these herbs into your diet, you can help improve your digestion and promote a healthier gut.

Another benefit of using herbs is their ability to reduce inflammation in the body. Chronic inflammation has been linked to a variety of health issues, such as heart disease, diabetes, and autoimmune disorders. Fortunately, many herbs have anti-inflammatory properties that can help reduce inflammation and promote overall health. Turmeric, for example, contains a compound called curcumin that has been found to be effective in fighting inflammation. Other herbs like cinnamon, rosemary, and oregano also have anti-inflammatory effects that can benefit the body.

Mental health is also an important aspect of overall well-being, and herbs can play a role in promoting a healthy mind. Many herbs have been traditionally used to improve mood and reduce stress and anxiety.

Chamomile, for example, has a calming effect and can help promote relaxation and better sleep. Lemon balm and lavender are also known for their calming properties, making them great herbs for reducing stress and anxiety.

Herbs into your daily routine can have numerous benefits for your health. From boosting the immune system to improving digestion and reducing inflammation, herbs offer a natural and effective way to support the body. Additionally, many herbs also have mental health benefits, promoting relaxation and reducing stress. With so many different herbs to choose from, there is something for everyone to help improve their overall health and well-being.

The power of herbs takes center stage in this enlightening journey. Herbs, nature's ancient remedies, have been trusted allies in the quest for health and vitality throughout the centuries. Their ability to support and enhance the body's natural processes is nothing short of remarkable. From boosting immunity to calming inflammation, these natural plants offer a plethora of benefits that promote holistic well being. Take, for instance, the mighty echinacea, a trusted companion when cold and flu symptoms arise. Its ability to strengthen the immune system and reduce the severity of these ailments is well documented. Ginger, turmeric, and garlic join the ranks, each bringing their unique immune boosting properties to the forefront. Ginger, with its warming properties, soothes aching throats and calms nausea, while turmeric's active compound, curcumin, fights inflammation throughout the body. The digestive system also finds solace in herbs. Peppermint, with its refreshing nature, brings relief from bloating, gas, and nausea. Fennel and ginger, too, are digestive heroes, promoting stomach comfort and easing discomfort. For centuries, these herbs have been relied upon to aid digestion and enhance gut health, and their effectiveness continues to be celebrated today. But the benefits of herbs extend beyond the physical. Mental well-being is an integral part of the health journey, and herbs like chamomile, lemon balm, and lavender play a pivotal role in promoting a calm and relaxed mind. Their calming properties help reduce stress and anxiety, encouraging a good night's rest and a sense of tranquility. Incorporating these natural allies into one's daily routine is a powerful step towards self-care and wellness. Whether it's brewing a soothing cup of chamomile tea, adding a dash of turmeric to a morning smoothie, or growing a windowsill garden of peppermint and lavender, these herbs offer a simple yet effective way to support the body's natural balance and unlock a treasure trove of health benefits.

The ancient practice of herbal remedies takes on a new light as one delves into the world of nutrient deficiencies. Herbs, with their potent properties, step forward as nature's solution to combating various deficiencies that plague modern day individuals. Take, for instance, the mighty nettle, a herb that grows wild and proud, offering a bounty of benefits. When infused into tea or added to soups and stews, nettle leaves provide a rich source of iron, perfect for combating iron deficiency and boosting energy levels.

Nature's pharmacy also presents dandelion, a humble weed often overlooked, yet packed with vitamin C and potassium. Dandelion leaves and roots, when carefully prepared, offer a natural solution for those lacking these essential nutrients. The world of herbs also shines a light on the power of adaptogens, natural substances that help the body adapt to stress and bring balance. Herbs like ashwagandha and rhodiola take center stage, offering support for those with adrenal fatigue and helping to regulate cortisol levels. These herbal allies are a gentle reminder that nature holds the key to wellness, providing a calming influence in a fast paced world. Furthermore, the bright and vibrant turmeric, with its active compound curcumin, not only fights inflammation but also supports brain health, making it an ideal herb for those seeking cognitive support. The journey of herbal remedies is a captivating adventure, where nature's bounty provides solutions for a range of health concerns. With each herb offering unique benefits, one embarks on a path of discovery, harnessing the power of nature to address nutrient deficiencies and promote overall vitality.

See Chapter 11 for the best herbs for our body parts.

Chapter Four

INCREASING ENERGY LEVELS

Increasing energy levels is a goal that many people strive for, whether it's to keep up with a busy schedule or to simply feel healthier and more alert. However, with the daily demands of life, it can often feel like there's just not enough energy to go around. So, what can be done to boost energy levels and keep them sustained throughout the day? This is a question that has been widely debated and researched, with various theories and methods proposed. In this piece, we will explore the different ways to increase energy levels and provide a diverse range of perspectives on the topic.

From a scientific perspective, there are several factors that can contribute to low energy levels. These include sleep deprivation, poor nutrition, stress, and lack of physical activity. Therefore, one of the most effective ways to increase energy levels is to address these underlying issues. Adequate sleep is essential for the body to recharge and rejuvenate, so getting 7-9 hours of quality sleep each night is crucial. Additionally, consuming f whole foods such as fruits, vegetables, nuts, seeds and healthy fats can provide the necessary nutrients for sustained energy. Regular exercise has also been proven to boost energy levels, as it helps to improve circulation, increase oxygen supply to the body, and release endorphins, which are natural mood and energy enhancers.

Aside from these lifestyle factors, there are also some natural remedies and practices that can help increase energy levels. One popular method is to incorporate adaptogenic herbs into one's diet. Adaptogens are a class of herbs that help the body adapt to stress and regulate its energy levels. Some examples of adaptogenic herbs include ashwagandha, ginseng, and rhodiola. Another practice that has gained traction in recent years is mindfulness meditation. By focusing on the present and calming the mind, meditation can help reduce stress and increase energy levels.

On the other hand, some people believe that increasing energy levels is not just about addressing physical and external factors, but also about tapping into one's inner energy reserves. This is where the concept of energy management comes into play. According to this perspective, energy is not a finite resource that needs to be constantly replenished, but rather a renewable one that can be managed and optimized. This can be achieved through activities such as prioritizing tasks, taking breaks, and setting boundaries to avoid burnout.

Others argue that the key to increasing energy levels lies in finding a sense of purpose and motivation. When one is passionate and driven about their goals and tasks, they are more likely to have high energy levels and feel fulfilled. This can be achieved by setting clear goals, practicing self care, and surrounding oneself with positive and supportive people.

There are various ways to increase energy levels, and the most effective approach may vary from person to person. Incorporating healthy habits such as getting enough sleep, eating well, and exercising regularly is essential. Additionally, incorporating natural remedies and practices, such as adaptogenic herbs and mindfulness meditation, can also have a positive impact. However, it's also crucial to consider the importance of energy management and finding purpose and motivation. By taking a holistic approach and addressing both external and internal factors, one can boost their energy levels and lead a more fulfilling and energetic life.

Chapter Five

THE POWER OF FRUIT

Fruits are an essential part of a healthy diet and have been proven to provide numerous benefits to the body. They are packed with vitamins, minerals, and antioxidants that are crucial for maintaining good health and improving overall performance.

One of the main benefits of fruits is their ability to boost the immune system. Fruits such as oranges, strawberries, and kiwis are rich in vitamin C, which is known to strengthen the immune system and protect the body against illnesses and infections. This is especially important for athletes and individuals who engage in high performance activities, as a strong immune system can help prevent them from getting sidelined by illnesses.

Moreover, fruits are also known to improve energy levels and enhance physical performance. They are a great source of natural sugars, which provide a quick burst of energy that is needed for physical activities. Additionally, fruits contain essential electrolytes like potassium and magnesium, which are crucial for maintaining proper muscle function and preventing cramps and fatigue during exercise.

In terms of impact on the body, fruits have been linked to numerous health benefits. Regular consumption of fruits has been shown to reduce the risk of chronic diseases such as heart disease, diabetes, and certain types of cancer. This is due to the high levels of antioxidants found in fruits, which help fight against free radicals and protect the body from oxidative stress.

It is important to note that the benefits of fruits are not limited to physical health. Fruits also have a positive impact on mental well-being. Studies have shown that individuals who consume a diet rich in fruits have lower levels of stress and better cognitive function.

In conclusion, the power of fruits cannot be underestimated. They provide numerous benefits to the body, including boosting the immune system, improving energy levels and physical performance, and protecting against chronic diseases. Incorporating a variety of fruits into our daily diet can have a significant impact on our overall health and well being.

There are numerous benefits to home juicing, both for overall health and for athletic performance. Juicing at home allows individuals to consume a variety of fresh fruits and vegetables in a convenient and easily digestible form. This can lead to increased energy levels, improved digestion, and a stronger immune system. Additionally, the high concentration of vitamins, minerals, and antioxidants in fresh juice can support healthy skin, hair, and nails. For athletes, this can translate to quicker recovery times, enhanced muscle repair, and improved endurance.

One of the main impacts of home juicing on the body is its ability to provide a quick and efficient source of nutrients. When fruits and vegetables are juiced, the fibrous pulp is removed, making the nutrients more readily available for absorption. This means that the body can quickly access the essential vitamins, minerals, and antioxidants to support its daily functions and repair any damage caused by physical exertion. This can be especially beneficial for athletes who require a higher intake of nutrients to support their active lifestyle.

The term "h302" is often used in the context of home juicing, and it refers to the section of the Hazard

Communication Standard (HCS) that outlines the potential health effects of chemicals. In the context of juicing, this term can be seen as a reminder to be mindful of the ingredients used in the juicing process and to prioritize organic and pesticide free produce. This can have a significant impact on the overall health benefits of home juicing, as consuming chemical free juice can help reduce the risk of potential negative health effects and ensure that the body receives only pure and beneficial nutrients.

Home juicing can have a significant impact on athletic performance and overall health. Its ability to provide a concentrated source of nutrients can support the body's functions and help individuals reach their fitness goals. However, it is important to consider the quality of ingredients and to maintain a balanced and varied diet to reap the full benefits of home juicing.

Washing Fruit

There are several methods for washing fruits and removing chemicals, and opinions may vary on which method is best. Some people prefer using a vinegar solution to wash their fruits, while others believe in using baking soda and alkalizing fruit. Baking soda is known for its cleaning properties and can effectively remove dirt, wax, and chemicals from the surface of fruits. To use this method, mix one teaspoon of baking soda with two cups of water and stir until the baking soda dissolves completely. Then, soak the fruits in the solution for a few minutes before rinsing them with clean water. This method is safe, easy, and cost effective.

On the other hand, some individuals believe that alkalizing fruits can also help eliminate chemicals. This method involves soaking the fruits in a bowl of water with a pH level of 8 or higher, which can be achieved by adding a few drops of lemon juice or apple cider vinegar. The theory behind this method is that the alkaline solution will neutralize any acidic or chemical residue on the fruits, making them safer to consume. However, there is limited scientific evidence to support this claim.

Ultimately, the best way to wash fruits and get rid of chemicals may depend on personal preference. Both baking soda and alkalizing fruits can be effective methods for removing chemicals, but it is important to thoroughly rinse the fruits with clean water after using these methods. Additionally, buying organic or locally grown fruits can also reduce exposure to chemicals. Overall, it is important to prioritize food safety and choose a method that makes you feel comfortable and confident in the cleanliness of your fruits.

Chapter Six

DETOX AND CLEANSING

Parasites are organisms that live off of another living host, using its resources to survive and reproduce. They can cause a range of health issues, from digestive problems to fatigue and even serious diseases. While there are many different types of parasites, there are also many natural herbs that can be used to help cleanse and detox the body from these harmful organisms.

One of the best ways to detox and cleanse using herbs is through the use of anti-parasitic herbs. These herbs have been used for centuries to help rid the body of parasites and restore balance to the digestive system. Some common anti-parasitic herbs include garlic, wormwood, black walnut, clove, and oregano. These herbs have powerful anti-microbial properties that can help kill and expel parasites from the body.

Another effective way to detox and cleanse using herbs is by incorporating bitter herbs into your diet. Bitter herbs, such as dandelion, burdock, and milk thistle, stimulate the liver and gallbladder, helping to flush toxins and waste from the body. This can help improve digestion and overall health, as well as help eliminate parasites.

In addition to specific anti-parasitic and bitter herbs, there are also a variety of herbs that can help support and strengthen the immune system. A strong immune system is essential in fighting off parasites and preventing them from taking hold in the body. Some of these immune-boosting herbs include echinacea, astragalus, and ginger.

Along with incorporating these herbs into your diet, there are also certain herbal remedies that can be used to specifically target parasites. For example, a herbal tincture made with a combination of anti-parasitic herbs can be taken daily to help eliminate parasites from the body. Another option is to do a parasite cleanse using a combination of herbs, supplements, and dietary changes.

It is important to note that while herbs can be powerful allies in the fight against parasites, they may not be enough on their own. It is also important to address any underlying issues that may have caused the parasite infestation, such as poor hygiene or a weakened immune system. This may involve making lifestyle changes and seeking the guidance of a healthcare professional.

Using herbs to detox and cleanse the body from parasites is a natural and effective approach. By incorporating anti-parasitic, bitter, and immune-boosting herbs into your diet and utilizing herbal remedies specific to parasites, you can help support your body's natural defense against these harmful organisms. However, it is important to address the root causes of the parasite infestation and seek professional guidance for a comprehensive and sustainable approach to parasite prevention and elimination.

Oregano oil is a powerful antiparasitic and antifungal property that can help combat infections caused by parasites and candida. This is because oregano oil contains a compound called carvacrol, which has been shown to have strong antimicrobial effects. It is believed that carvacrol can disrupt the cell membranes of parasites and fungi, ultimately killing them.

There are several foods that have been found to have anti-parasitic properties and can help to naturally remove parasites from the body. One of the best foods for this purpose is garlic. Garlic contains a compound called allicin, which has been shown to have strong anti-parasitic effects. It can help to kill parasites and their eggs, while also boosting the immune system.

Papaya seeds are another great food for removing parasites. These seeds contain an enzyme called papain, which has been found to be effective against parasitic infections. Consuming papaya seeds can help to break down the protective outer layer of parasites, making them easier for the body to eliminate.

Pumpkin seeds are also known for their antiparasitic properties. They contain a compound called cucurbitacin, which has been found to paralyze parasites and prevent them from attaching to the intestinal wall. This makes it easier for the body to eliminate them.

Jalapeno Chile Peppers for removing parasites in the body. Some experts believe that the active compound in jalapenos, capsaicin, has antiparasitic properties that can help to kill or expel parasites from the body. Additionally, jalapenos are high in vitamin C, which can boost the immune system and help the body fight off parasitic infections. Furthermore, jalapenos are a source of fiber, which can aid in digestion and promote regular bowel movements, helping to flush out parasites from the digestive tract.

Walnuts are known for their numerous health benefits, and one of them is their ability to remove parasites from the body. This is due to the presence of certain compounds and nutrients in walnuts that have antiparasitic properties.

One such compound is juglone, which is found in the outer layer of the walnut's shell. Juglone has been shown to have strong anti-parasitic effects and can help eliminate parasites from the digestive tract. It does so by inhibiting the growth and reproduction of parasites, making it difficult for them to survive and thrive in the body. Additionally, walnuts are rich in omega-3 fatty acids, which have been found to have anti-inflammatory and immune-boosting properties. This helps strengthen the body's defenses against parasites and reduces the risk of infection.

In addition to these specific foods, a diet rich in fruits, vegetables, and whole grains can also help to naturally remove parasites. These foods provide essential vitamins, minerals, and antioxidants that support a healthy immune system, making it easier for the body to fight off and eliminate parasites.

Some proponents of oregano oil claim that it has powerful antiparasitic and antifungal properties that can help combat infections caused by parasites and candida. This is because oregano oil contains a compound called carvacrol, which has been shown to have strong antimicrobial effects. It is believed that carvacrol can disrupt the cell membranes of parasites and fungi, ultimately eliminating them.

Detoxing parasites from the body is a process that requires dedication and commitment. It involves cleansing the body of harmful organisms that can cause various health issues. To effectively detox parasites, a proper schedule needs to be followed. Here is a sample schedule that can help in the process.

It's essential to start with a healthy and balanced diet. This includes plenty of fresh fruits, vegetables, nuts and seeds, these foods contain essential nutrients that can support your body's detoxification process.

In addition to a healthy diet, incorporating garlic, ginger, cayenne pepper, cinnamon and turmeric can help to kill parasites and support the immune system. These can be taken in the form of added to meals or herbal teas.

To further aid in the detox process, it is crucial to limit or avoid processed and sugary foods. These foods can feed parasites and hinder the detoxification process. Drinking plenty of water and herbal teas can also help to flush out toxins from the body.

Regular exercise is also beneficial in detoxing parasites. It helps to improve blood circulation and support the body's natural detoxification systems. Engaging in activities such as yoga and deep breathing exercises can also help to reduce stress, which can strengthen the immune system and make the body more stronger.

Binders are an essential component of any parasite cleanse. The purpose of a binder is to help remove toxins and other harmful substances from the body. Parasite cleansing can release a significant amount of toxins into the body, and without a binder, these toxins can continue to circulate and cause harm. Binders work by binding to these toxins and helping to eliminate them from the body through the digestive system.

The frequency of taking a binder during a parasite cleanse will depend on the individual's specific needs. It is recommended to take a binder at least once a day during a cleanse, but some people may need to take it more frequently depending on their symptoms and the severity of their parasite infestation. It is important to listen to your body and adjust the frequency of binder intake accordingly.

When it comes to choosing the best binder for a parasite cleanse, there are several options available. Some popular binders include activated charcoal, bentonite clay, and chlorella. These binders are known for their ability to attract and absorb toxins.

Using a binder during a parasite cleanse is crucial for a successful and safe detoxification process. It helps to remove toxins and prevent them from causing harm to the body. The frequency of binder intake may vary from person to person, and it is important to choose a binder that suits your individual needs. Incorporating a binder into your parasite cleanse can help ensure a thorough and effective detoxification.

Overall, detoxing parasites requires a holistic approach that includes a healthy diet, Herbs, exercise, and consistency. It is also important to keep in mind that every individual's body is different, and the detox process may vary. Therefore, it is essential to listen to your body and adjust the schedule accordingly. With dedication and patience, a successful parasite detox can lead to improved overall health and well-being.

Lastly, it is crucial to maintain consistency and follow the detox schedule for at least 4-6 weeks. This allows enough time for the body to eliminate parasites and heal from any damage caused by them. A break of 2 weeks access and see if they have all been eliminated, if not then repeat the cycle

Chapter Seven

FASTING

Fasting is the practice of abstaining from food and sometimes drink for a specified period of time. It has been used for centuries as a spiritual or religious practice in many cultures, but in recent years has gained popularity as a health and wellness tool. There are many different types of fasting, ranging from intermittent fasting, where one cycles between periods of eating and fasting, to extended fasts lasting multiple days.

Fasting has been linked to a range of health benefits, including weight loss, improved digestion, increased energy levels, and even a longer lifespan. The underlying principle of fasting is that by giving the digestive system a break, the body is able to focus on other essential processes, such as repairing cells and regulating hormones. Additionally, periods of fasting can also lead to a process called autophagy, where the body breaks down and recycles damaged cells, potentially reducing the risk of chronic diseases.

So, how does one implement fasting into their lifestyle? The first step is to understand the different types of fasting and choose the one that best suits your goals and lifestyle. Some popular methods include:

1. Intermittent fasting: This involves cycling between periods of eating and fasting. It can range from a daily schedule of 16 hours of fasting and 8 hours of eating, to a more extreme approach of 24 hours of fasting and only one meal per day.

2. Water fasting: This involves consuming only water for a designated period of time, usually lasting between 24 hours to several days.

3. Juice fasting: This involves consuming only fresh juices, water, and herbal teas for a designated period of time, typically ranging from 1-3 days.

4. Modified fasting: This approach involves consuming a limited amount of calories on fasting days, usually around 500-600 calories,

while still restricting food intake for a designated period of time.

Once you have chosen a fasting method, it is important to gradually build up the hours or days of fasting. For example, if you are new to fasting, you may want to start with intermittent fasting and gradually increase the fasting period from 12 hours to 16 hours. It is important to listen to your body and not push yourself too hard. It may also be beneficial to consult with a healthcare professional before starting any type of fasting regimen.

It is also important to have a plan for breaking your fast. After a period of fasting, the body may have a sensitive digestive system, so it is important to reintroduce food slowly and mindfully. Start with easily digestible foods such as soups, smoothies, and fruits, and gradually incorporate more solid foods.

When it comes to the duration of fasting, it is important to find a balance that works for you. Some people may benefit from shorter fasts, while others may see more benefits from longer fasts. It is also important to listen to your body and end the fast if you are feeling weak, dizzy, or unwell.

Breaking a fast refers to the process of ending a period of abstaining from food and possibly other activities. How one breaks a fast can vary depending on factors such as the duration of the fast, the individual's health and dietary needs, and cultural or religious practices. One common approach to breaking a fast is to start with small, easily digestible meals and gradually increase the size and complexity of the meals over a period of several days.

Some may choose to break a fast with a light meal, such as a bowl of vegetable broth or a piece of fruit, before gradually incorporating more substantial foods. It is also important to stay hydrated by drinking plenty of water throughout the day. Additionally, it is recommended to avoid heavy or greasy foods, as they may cause discomfort or digestive issues after a period of fasting.

Others may prefer to break their fast with a larger meal, especially if the fast has been shorter in duration. In this case, it is still important to start with easily digestible foods and gradually introduce more complex and heavier foods.

When it comes to the timing of breaking a fast, some may choose to break their fast in the morning with breakfast, while others may prefer to break their fast in the evening with dinner. Again, this may depend on personal preference and individual circumstances.

It is always important to listen to your body and pay attention to any discomfort or changes in digestion when breaking a fast. If any issues arise, it is best to consult a healthcare professional for guidance. Overall, the key is to approach breaking a fast mindfully and with intention, gradually reintroducing food and listening to the body's needs.

In conclusion, fasting can be a beneficial practice for both spiritual and physical health. It is important to choose a fasting method that fits your goals and lifestyle, gradually build up the hours or days of fasting, and have a plan for breaking the fast. Remember to listen to your body and consult with a healthcare professional before starting any fasting regimen. With proper implementation and understanding, fasting can be a powerful tool for improving overall health and well-being.

Chapter Eight

MINERALS AND COPPER WATER

There is no denying the importance of minerals in our diets. These essential micronutrients play a crucial role in maintaining overall health and well-being. From building strong bones and teeth to regulating our metabolism and supporting immune function, minerals are vital for our bodies to function properly.

One of the key benefits of consuming foods rich in minerals is their role in maintaining strong bones and teeth. Calcium, phosphorus, and magnesium are all essential minerals for bone health and help prevent conditions like osteoporosis. Additionally, minerals like potassium and sodium help regulate the fluid balance in our bodies, which is essential for maintaining healthy blood pressure levels.

Minerals also play a significant role in our metabolism. Iron, for example, is essential for the production of red blood cells, which carry oxygen throughout our bodies. Zinc is another mineral that aids in metabolism by helping enzymes break down food and assisting in the production of hormones.

Furthermore, minerals are crucial for supporting our immune system. Selenium, zinc, and copper are all essential minerals that help our bodies fight off infections and diseases. These minerals also play a role in wound healing and tissue repair.

While minerals are found in a variety of foods, it is essential to consume a diverse and balanced diet to ensure adequate intake. Dark leafy greens, nuts, seeds, legumes, and whole grains are all excellent sources of minerals. However, it is crucial to note that certain factors like soil quality, food processing, and cooking methods can affect the mineral content in our food.

The importance of minerals in our diets cannot be overstated. From maintaining bone health to supporting our metabolism and immune system, these micronutrients play a crucial role in keeping our bodies functioning at their best. Therefore, it is essential to make an effort to include a variety of mineral rich foods in our diets to reap their numerous benefits.

Drinking copper water has been a practice for centuries, and for good reason. Copper is an essential mineral that plays a crucial role in maintaining overall health and well-being. When water is stored in a copper vessel, tiny particles of copper leach into the water, enriching it with its numerous health benefits.

One of the main benefits of drinking copper water is its ability to boost the immune system. Copper is known for its antibacterial, antiviral and antiinflammatory properties, making it an effective remedy for fighting off infections and illnesses. It also aids in the production of white blood cells, which are responsible for fighting off foreign invaders in the body.

Another advantage of drinking copper water is its ability to improve digestion. Copper helps to stimulate the digestive enzymes, promoting better digestion and absorption of nutrients. It also helps to cleanse and detoxify the stomach, ensuring a healthy gut and preventing digestive issues like constipation, bloating, and gas.

Furthermore, copper water is believed to have anti-aging properties. Copper is a powerful antioxidant that helps to fight free radicals and prevent cell damage, keeping the skin youthful and radiant. It also aids in the production of collagen, a protein that keeps the skin firm and supple.

Apart from its numerous benefits to the body, drinking copper water also has an impact on the human electric field. Copper is a good conductor of electricity, and it is believed that drinking copper water can help to balance the body's natural electric field. This can result in better energy levels, improved mood, and increased focus and concentration.

However, it is important to note that drinking copper water should be done in moderation. Too much copper in the body can lead to copper toxicity, which can cause serious health issues. It is recommended to drink one glass of copper water per day to reap its benefits without any adverse effects.

Drinking copper water has numerous benefits for the body, including boosting the immune system, improving digestion, and promoting anti-aging effects. It also has a positive impact on the human electric field. However, it is essential to be mindful of the amount of copper water consumed to avoid any potential risks.

Chapter Nine

MEDITATION

Meditation has been practiced for thousands of years and has been shown to have numerous benefits for both the mind and body. It is a technique that involves training the mind to focus and redirect thoughts, leading to a state of calmness and relaxation. The benefits of meditation range from reducing stress and anxiety to improving emotional well-being and overall health.

One of the main benefits of meditation is its ability to reduce stress and anxiety. By focusing on the present moment and quieting the mind, meditation can help individuals let go of worries and concerns, leading to a sense of calmness and peace. This can be particularly helpful for those who struggle with chronic stress or anxiety disorders.

In addition to reducing stress, meditation has been shown to improve emotional well-being. Regular practice of meditation can help individuals develop a greater sense of self-awareness and self-acceptance. This can lead to improved mood and a more positive outlook on life.

Meditation also has physical benefits, such as lowering blood pressure and boosting the immune system. By reducing stress and promoting relaxation, meditation can have a positive impact on overall health and wellness.

Implementing meditation into daily life can be done in a variety of ways. Some popular methods include sitting in a quiet place and focusing on the breath, repeating a mantra or phrase, or participating in guided meditation sessions. It is important to find a method that works best for you and to make it a regular practice to reap the full benefits.

Meditation is a practice that allows individuals to connect with their inner selves and the divine consciousness. It is a way to quiet the mind, let go of distractions and focus on the present moment. Through meditation, we can tap into our spiritual nature and tap into the universal energy that connects us all.

There are various forms of meditation, but the ultimate goal is the same to achieve a state of peace, calmness, and unity with the divine. Some people use breathing techniques, mantras, or visualization to aid in their meditation practice. Others may choose to focus on a particular object or simply observe their thoughts without judgment.

Regardless of the method, meditation can bring about a sense of clarity, inner peace, and a deeper understanding of oneself and the world around us. It allows us to detach from our external surroundings and connect with our true essence.

Through meditation, we can access the divine consciousness that exists within all of us. This universal energy is a source of infinite wisdom, love, and guidance. By quieting our minds and opening our hearts, we can receive insights, inspiration, and healing from the divine.

In today's fast-paced world, meditation is becoming increasingly important as a way to find inner balance and peace amidst the chaos. It is a powerful tool that can help us navigate through life with more clarity, purpose, and connection to the divine. As we continue to deepen our meditation practice, we can experience a profound sense of oneness with the universe and our true selves.

Chapter Ten

GROUNDING AND SUN GAZING

Grounding, also known as earthing, is the practice of connecting to the earth's surface by walking barefoot or using grounding devices such as mats or patches. The earth's surface has a negative charge, and when we make direct contact with it, it can help neutralize the positive charge in our bodies. This process has been shown to have numerous benefits, including balancing the body's pH level.

The pH level refers to the level of acidity or alkalinity in the body. A balanced pH level is essential for overall health and wellbeing, as it affects all bodily functions. The human body has a natural pH level of around 7.4, which is slightly alkaline. However, due to factors such as stress, pollution, and poor nutrition, our bodies can become more acidic.

When we are grounded, the earth's negative charge can help balance the positive charge in our bodies. This, in turn, can help regulate our pH level and bring it back to a more alkaline state. This is important because an overly acidic body can lead to various health issues, such as inflammation, digestive problems, and weakened immune system.

Moreover, grounding has also been shown to reduce stress and promote relaxation, which can also positively impact our pH level. When we are stressed, our bodies produce more acid, leading to an imbalance in our pH level. By reducing stress through grounding, we can help maintain a healthy pH level and prevent potential health problems.

In addition to grounding, maintaining a balanced and alkaline diet can also help regulate our pH level. Eating foods such as fruits, vegetables, and whole grains can help keep our bodies alkaline. However, in today's fast paced and processed food culture, it can be challenging to maintain a balanced diet. Therefore, incorporating grounding into our daily lives can be a simple and effective way to help balance our pH level and promote overall health and well-being.

Staring directly at the sun during specific periods of the day, such as the break of dawn or the falling of dusk, is a customary ritual known as sun gazing. This age old method has been employed by diverse societies over centuries and has recently gained traction due to its potential health benefits. One of the key advantages of sun gazing is its positive impact on the eyes. By exposing the eyes to the sun's radiance, it can enhance visual acuity and diminish the risk of ocular ailments like cataracts and macular degeneration. The sun's beams also invigorate the production of melatonin, a hormone that regulates the sleep wake cycle and can promote overall ocular wellness. Additionally, it is believed that sun gazing stimulates the pineal gland, which is responsible for generating melatonin and regulating other hormones in the body. This can lead to improved sleep, heightened energy levels, and a fortified immune system. In conclusion, sun gazing holds the potential to yield numerous advantages for both the eyes and the body, making it a valuable practice for overall well-being and health.

Chapter Eleven

HERBS FOR THE BODY

Below you can find a list of some of the best herbs for our body parts.

Brain

1. Ginkgo Biloba

2. Bacopa Monnieri

3. Ashwagandha

4. Rosemary

5. Turmeric

6. Sage

7. Ginseng

8. Gotu Kola

9. Lion's Mane Mushroom

10. Rhodiola Rosea

Eyes

1. Bilberry:

2. Ginkgo Biloba

3. Eyebright

4. Turmeric

5. Fennel

6. Saffron

7. Rosemary

8. Calendula

9. Green tea

10. Aloe vera

Sinuses

1. Echinacea

2. Goldenseal

3. Peppermint

4. Garlic

5. Horseradish

6. Ginger

7. Turmeric

8. Nettle

9. Elderberry

10. Licorice

Immune System

1. Echinacea

2. Astragalus

3. Reishi mushrooms

4. Elderberry

5. Garlic

6. Ginger

7. Turmeric

8. Cat's claw

9. Olive leaf

10. Ashwagandha

11. Licorice root

12. Andrographis

13. Holy basil

14. Oregano

15. Green tea

16. Rosemary

17. Sage

18. Thyme

19. Tulsi

20. Chamomile

Lungs

1. Mullein

2. Eucalyptus

3. Thyme

4. Licorice Root

5. Oregano

6. Ginger

7. Peppermint

8. Marshmallow Root

9. Ginseng

10. Lobelia

Liver

1. Milk thistle

2. Dandelion root

3. Turmeric

4. Artichoke

5. Schisandra

6. Burdock root

7. Licorice root

8. Chicory root

9. Reishi mushroom

10. Green tea

Pancreases

1. Turmeric

2. Holy basil

3. Milk thistle

4. Dandelion root

5. Licorice root

6. Ginger

7. Cinnamon

8. Rosemary

9. Oregano

10. Ginseng

11. Aloe vera

12. Peppermint

13. Chamomile

14. Fennel

15. Garlic

Heart

1. Garlic

2. Hawthorn

3. Ginger

4. Turmeric

5. Cinnamon

6. Cayenne pepper

7. Green tea

8. Holy basil

9. Arjuna

10. Ginkgo biloba

Kidneys And Adrenal Glands

1. Dandelion root

2. Ginger

3. Turmeric

4. Nettle leaf

5. Parsley

6. Marshmallow root

7. Chanca piedra

8. Corn silk

9. Buchu

10. Rehmannia

11. Rosemary

12. Licorice root

13. Astragalus

14. Cinnamon

15. Milk thistle.

Lymphatic System

1. Cleavers

2. Red clover

3. Burdock root

4. Echinacea

5. Goldenseal

6. Astragalus

7. Ginger

8. Dandelion root

9. Milk thistle

10. Calendula

Skin

1. Aloe Vera

2. Rosemary

3. Calendula

4. Chamomile

5. Peppermint

6. Neem

7. Comfrey

8. Echinacea

9. Red Clover

10. Nettle.

Nervous System

1. Ashwagandha

2. Skullcap

3. Passionflower

4. Valerian

5. Lemon balm

6. Rhodiola

7. Chamomile

8. Kava

9. Holy basil

10. Gotu kola

Intestines And Bowels

1. Peppermint

2. Fennel

3. Ginger

4. Slippery elm

5. Aloe vera

6. Chamomile

7. Turmeric

8. Dandelion

9. Marshmallow root

10. Licorice root

Joints

1. Turmeric

2. Ginger

3. Comfrey

4. Devil's Claw

5. Cat's Claw

6. Willow Bark

7. Ashwagandha

8. Eucalyptus

9. Stinging Nettle

10. Licorice Root

Ways to prepare Herbs:

Tips for Simmering Herbs:

1. Use fresh herbs whenever possible for the best flavor and potency.

2. Use a ratio of 1 tablespoon of herbs to 1 cup of water.

3. Crush or bruise the herbs before simmering to release their oils and flavors.

4. Keep the heat on low to prevent the herbs from burning or losing their potency.

5. You can add other ingredients like spices, fruits, or honey to enhance the flavor of your herbal infusion.

Tips for Warming Herbs:

1. Use dried herbs for warming as they tend to have a stronger flavor.

2. Use a ratio of 1 teaspoon of herbs to 1 cup of liquid (oil, water, alcohol).

3. Warm the herbs for 30 seconds to a minute at a time to prevent them from burning.

4. Stir the herbs occasionally to ensure they are evenly warmed.

5. After warming, let the herbs sit for a few minutes to allow the flavors to fully develop before using them

Cold Water Infusion:

1. Fresh herbs: The best way to prepare fresh herbs for infusing cold water is to thoroughly

wash and dry them before adding them to the water. You can leave the herbs whole or chop them up into smaller pieces for better flavor infusion.

2. Dried herbs: Dried herbs can also be used for infusing cold water, but they may take longer to release their flavors. You can either use whole dried herbs or crush them slightly before adding them to the water.

3. Fruits and vegetables: Adding slices of fresh fruits and vegetables can enhance the flavor of your infused water. Wash and cut the fruits and vegetables into small pieces before adding them to the water.

4. Citrus fruits: Citrus fruits like lemons, limes, and oranges are great for infusing cold water. Simply slice them and add them to the water for a refreshing and tangy flavor.

5. Berries: Berries are another great addition to infused water. Crush them slightly to release their juices and add them to the water for a burst of flavor.

6. Herbs and fruit combinations: Get creative and try different combinations of herbs and

fruits to find your favorite flavor. Some popular combinations include mint and cucumber, basil and strawberry, and rosemary and lemon.

7. Let it sit: Once you have added the herbs and fruits to the water, let it sit in the fridge for at least 2-4 hours or overnight for maximum flavor infusion.

8. Filter the water: If you are using tap water, it is best to filter it before infusing it with herbs. This will ensure that your water is free from any impurities and chemicals.

9. Use a pitcher or bottle with a filter: To make it convenient, you can use a pitcher or water bottle with a built-in filter to infuse your water. This will save you the hassle of straining out the herbs and fruits later.

10. Enjoy it cold: Infused water tastes best when served chilled. You can add ice cubes to your pitcher or bottle to keep it cool and refreshing.

Chapter Twelve

SETTING GOALS AND ENJOYING THE JOURNEY

Setting goals is an essential aspect of personal and professional development. It allows individuals to have a clear direction in life and motivates them to work towards achieving their desired outcomes. The process of setting and pursuing goals can be challenging, but it also brings numerous benefits and a sense of fulfillment.

One of the main benefits of setting goals is that it gives individuals a sense of purpose and direction. When we have a clear goal in mind, we are more likely to stay focused and motivated in our daily lives. It helps us prioritize our tasks and make decisions that align with our objectives, leading to a sense of satisfaction.

Moreover, setting goals also allows individuals to challenge themselves and push their limits. When we have a specific target to achieve, we are more likely to step out of our comfort zone and take risks. This not only helps us grow as individuals but also opens up new opportunities and experiences. Whether it is personal or professional goals, the process of working towards them helps us become more resilient, adaptable, and confident.

In addition to personal growth, setting goals also leads to improved productivity and efficiency. When we have a clear goal, we are more likely to plan and prioritize our tasks effectively. This not only helps us manage our time more efficiently but also ensures that we are working towards meaningful and achievable outcomes. As a result, we can accomplish more in less time and achieve a sense of accomplishment.

Furthermore, setting goals also helps individuals develop a growth mindset. Instead of being fixated on the end result, individuals who set goals focus on the process and see challenges as opportunities for learning and growth. This mindset allows individuals to develop resilience, problem solving skills, and the ability to adapt to changing circumstances. As a result, individuals become more confident in their abilities and can overcome setbacks and obstacles more effectively.